FORGIVENESS IS THERAPEUTIC

DR. TANDY NANCE AND
D. SHAHID

About The Authors

As the Founder and CEO of Redesign Your Life, LLC. Dr.Tandy Nance is a highly accomplished and dedicated Metaphysician, Certified Holistic Life Coach, International Author, and motivational Speaker. With over 18 years of experience in the mental health field, Dr. Tandy has amassed an impressive array of academic qualifications, including a Bachelor's degree in Criminal Justice, a Master's degree in Counseling Studies, a Master's degree in Business Administration, and a Doctorate in Metaphysical Humanistic Science.

Dr. Tandy is also the self-published author of "The Diva Code" a guide to leveling up designed to encourage self-improvement, the motivational self-help book "Boundaries+Clarity=Peace" which is designed to assist individuals who are struggling to create boundaries and gain the clarity necessary to make positive changes in their lives, "Your Body Is Your Castle" a six-week guide to eating healthier and having a positive body image, and co-author of "Forgiveness Is Therapeutic" created to emphasize the power of forgiveness, healing, and moving forward. Her books aim to empower people to find peace and fulfillment in their lives.

 D. Shahid is a throwback native New Yorker. He is committed to change, rehabilitation, and evolution. D. Shahid is the co-founder of the Heart of a Hustla brand, and Co-Owner of Heart of a H.U.S.T.L.A. Publishing.
D. Shahid is dedicated to changing the negative connotations attached to the term Hustla. H.U.S.T.L.A. is an acronym that represents:
H. HAVING
U. UNDYING
S. STRENGTH
T. TO
L. LEVITATE
A. ABOVE
Levitating above any obstacle that life may throw at you is his definition of what a Hustla truly is. D. Shahid is the epitome of the term H.U.S.T.L.A. He himself has levitated and overcome lifestyle choices that cost him 20 years of his life. He Has Undying Strength to levitate above because he is the true definition of a H.U.S.T.L.A.

Copyright Page

Copyright © 2023 Dr. Tandy Nance

Dedication

D. Shahid would like to dedicate this book to his
Queen Chevi, his rocks
Jay, Zay, Ken, Sam, and his father Cornell Gaskin may
you continue to rest in peace.

I would like to dedicate this book to my favorite Aunt
Betty and Aunt Barbra. May you continue to rest in
peace.

I also would like to thank D. Shahid for sharing this
experience with me. You are a part of my forgiveness
journey and I appreciate you.
-Dr. Tandy

INTRODUCTION

Welcome to "Forgiveness Is Therapeutic". A compelling book on the power of forgiveness. Forgiveness can sometimes be a difficult journey to start and is a process that takes time. In order to start forgiving you must make a conscious effort to let go of hurtful events by releasing negative thought patterns, anger, resentment, and pain. And also making an active choice to no longer suffer from the harm that was done to you.

Anger and resentment will keep you stuck in the past overcome by disempowering emotions, instead of living in the present. Forgiveness is a commitment to change, and it takes practice. If you're struggling with starting your forgiveness journey, today you will find the answers that will help you overcome the anger and pain, and move toward the healing process. This book will help you prepare for your journey by showing you how to be honest with yourself, vulnerable, and aware of all the things you need to start your forgiveness journey. All I ask is that you keep an open mind and an open heart.

Dr. Tandy

"It's not an easy journey, to get to a place where you forgive people. But it is such a powerful place because it frees you."

Tyler Perry

But one thing I do:forgetting what is behind,and pressing toward that which is ahead.

PHILIPPIANS 3:13

Part 1
Everything Starts With Self

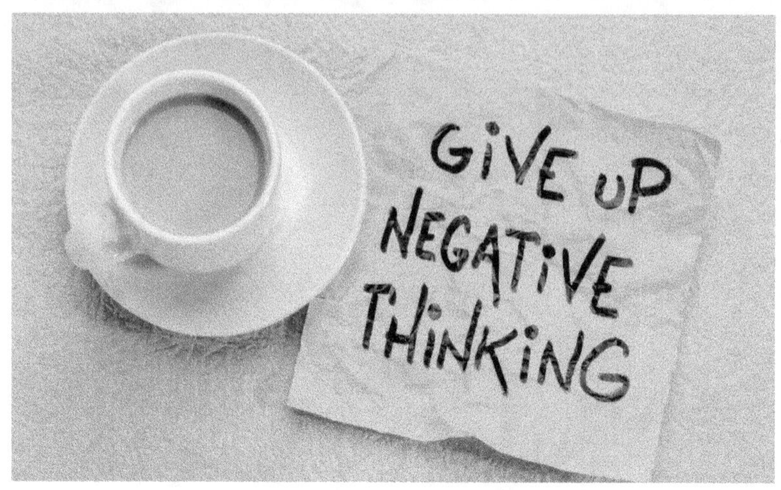

The Power of Thought

Holding on to unforgiveness keeps us living in the past. It stifles our growth and anchors us. This anchor prevents us from moving forward in life as it tethers us to unhappiness, unstableness, and mediocrity. One's ultimate goal of peace, love, and happiness is unachievable because of this anchor. It is only attainable once we develop the gift of forgiveness. Forgiveness propels us toward the three goals of peace, love, and happiness.

"We must develop and maintain the capacity to forgive. He who is devoid of the power to forgive is devoid of the power to love."
-Martin Luther King Jr.

Oftentimes in life, we get overwhelmed. It may seem like we are getting hit from every side As we are blown to and from. Life can be brutal, and it is during these times that we may play the blame game. This is very typical. Most people blame-shift by blaming others. The other group of people blame-shift by blaming themselves. Either way, blame is cast. It's even suggested that the people who blame themselves are being responsible. This could be the case, but the fallout is the same. This is indeed a fragile thing. Self-blame if not careful, can turn into self-loathing and self-hate. Self-loathing and self-hate translate to the un-forgiveness of oneself. This is the worst kind of unforgiveness. Unforgiveness of self.

The Yoke of unforgiveness affects us either physically, mentally, or spiritually. Unforgiveness is like a cancer. If left unchecked, unforgiveness turns into anger. John HopkinsMedicine.org states that there are physical effects of not forgiving someone. "ChronicAnger puts you into a fight or flight mode, which results in numerous changes in your body. These changes can be in heart rate, blood pressure, and immune response. Those changes then increase the risk of depression, heart disease, and diabetes, among other conditions". Forgiveness however calms stress levels which leads to improved health.

 Unforgiveness also affects us mentally. Hopkins medicine.org states:" People who tend to hold grudges, however, are more likely to experience severe depression and post-traumatic stress disorder, as well as other health conditions ". WWW.health.harvard.edu states:" Practicing forgiveness can have powerful health benefits. Observational studies, and even some randomized trials, suggest that forgiveness is associated with lower levels of depression, anxiety, and hostility; Reduced substance abuse; higher self-esteem; and greater life satisfaction". So as stated thus far Unforgiveness affects us negatively physically and mentally. Forgiveness on the other hand affects both our physical and mental state positively. However, it doesn't end there. Unforgiveness also affects us spiritually as well.

Unforgiveness is like a tourniquet that stops the flow of God's blessing in our lives. The term 'God don't bless mess' is alive here. Unforgiveness is equivalent to the mess. A stew or witches brew that creates separation from the Divine. Bellevue Christian counseling states:" Unforgiveness affects your spirit and your soul, hindering your spiritual growth and fruitfulness. You may feel spiritually dry, stuck, or stalled in your spiritual life. Unforgiveness builds a wall between you and God. Fear replaces peace and imprisonment replaces freedom". The only way to be set free from that spiritual bondage is to repent and ask for forgiveness.

So in this, you can see the power of forgiveness and the destruction of unforgiveness. Forgiveness is a powerful tool that if used properly can elevate us to a life of utopic proportions.

So as we can see unforgiveness affects us in three areas of our lives. It affects us physically mentally and spiritually. We have to identify where we are lacking. We have to be honest with ourselves. We have to look at our lives and identify where we were unforgiving, either to ourselves or to others. Once we identify the toxic trait of unforgiveness, we must flip the switch from unforgiven to forgiving. The pitfalls of unforgiveness, the muck and mire of unforgiveness, and the Fallout of unforgiveness can and will affect us all. No one is above it, and it is no respecter of man. The hardest person to forgive sometimes is yourself. We are our hardest judge at times. We can be our worst critic. The spirit of unworthiness, doubt, self-hatred, low self-esteem, pettiness, and no self-worth to name a few, are all born from us not being able to forgive self. One begets the other like a domino effect. These negative identifiers are dream crushers, and people destroyers. If not careful it can sap all of the goodness out of us, and leave us as a shell of our former self. It can consume us with unhappiness and gloom. If left unchecked the after-effects of Unforgiveness can invade all of our thoughts.

THOUGHT(Thot) n.1 The product of mental activity. 2. An idea or notion. 3. The act or process of thinking. 4. The capacity, or faculty of thinking. 5. Consideration or attention. 6. An opinion, or belief.
-Randall House

Before any form of action, before any word, and before any deed, there is first the spark. The spark of which I am speaking of is called thought. The embodiment of thought should go through a refining process that is rooted in Forgiveness. Thought from its embryonic to its born stage; however long the process, is the force that is necessary in order to manifest all. The spark(thought) once ignited brings to life anything, and everything imaginable.

The gift, and power of thought aren't a problem. In all actuality, it is a blessing. The curse, or problem of thought, only comes into play when we're not thinking, visualizing, and imagining positive things. The pitfalls of thought rest in the negativity that exists in our state of Unforgiveness. This Poisonous mind frame must be overcome and abolished. We have a negative side within us, and a positive side within us. This is called the duality of man. Good and evil both co-exist within ourselves(the mind). We must strive to keep our thoughts righteous, divine, pure, and refined in order to build and maintain a positive magnetic field that promotes the state of forgiveness.

So we must protect our thoughts. We have to keep our thoughts positive, pristine, and forward. Holding on to resentment keeps us living in the past. Thought equals view. So if we view ourselves as Worthy, we will begin to think that we are worthy. Unforgiveness dwells in "stinkin' thinkin' ". I'm not worth it. I'm a loser. It's all my fault. I'm a failure, a bum, and thinking along those lines is stinkin' thinkin'.

The longer we spend in positive thought, the brighter that spark will be. The stronger, and Sounder the thought, the better we'll be equipped in order to bring the thought to fruition. Manifestation of the thought is the active process of putting the thought into motion. The power lies in the thought. "As a man thinketh so he shall be in his heart." -proverbs 23:7 I am a king. I am a queen. I am a winner. I am somebody. I can do it. I am worthy. I am blessed. I am driven. I am forgiven. My future is bright. Thinking along these lines leads to a life filled with happiness, and achieved goals.

You have the power within to build your own reality. You are the master builder. Before any builder can bring his/her blueprints to life, He/She has to have a thought. Good righteous forgiving thoughts equals skyscrapers. Stinkin' thinkin' unforgiving thoughts equal destruction and a life in shambles. Utilize the spirit of forgiveness. It is therapeutic, and it will assist you in being a master builder.

A sense of peace will usher its way in and grant you the clarity needed to build.

Do not underestimate, or minimize the power of thought. Think right, and get right. Guard your thoughts, and reduce your intake of idleness. We can be whatever it is we think we can become. It sounds so simple, but it's not so easy. Familiarity creeps in. The old familiar spirits of insecurity, unbelief, doubt, and Unforgiveness creep in and rob us of a bright productive existence. We slide back in thought instead of forward thinking.

Once we change the thoughts that we have of ourselves, the new thoughts will make way for evolution. The negative thought will turn into a positive thought, and unforgiveness will turn into forgiveness. "Be careful what you think, because your thoughts run your life." -Proverbs 4:23 This is a process. As Dr.Tandy will discuss later, you have to trust the process.

Some are under the illusion that the graduation process of evolution from unforgiveness to forgiveness is an automatic one. This is the furthest from the truth. It takes hard work, repetition, and continuity. You cannot erase years of negative thinking overnight. It is impossible. You have to put in the work with positive reinforcements such as groups, therapy, coaching, and surrounding yourself with like-minded individuals, and you have to be committed. Pessimism to optimism takes wisdom. This wisdom comes about by applying the knowledge that you've learned. This means you have to think it, then live it.

The newfound knowledge of the forgiven you has to be lived. You have to walk in your new purpose. This takes practice, practice, practice! At the first storm in life you cannot revert back to the unforgiven you. You have been redeemed. Walk in your Redemption. After you unpack all the negative things that caused your initial way of living an unforgiving life, you must repack with whatever will remind you that you are now living a life of forgiveness. A forgiven life is a fruitful and productive life, and it is sparked by THOUGHT.

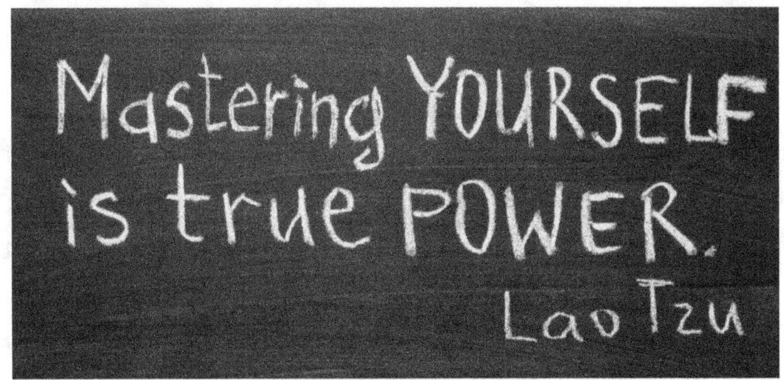

THE ULTIMATE FORGIVENESS

Self-forgiveness is the most important type of forgiveness. If you cannot forgive yourself, you are not capable of forgiving anyone else. It's just like love. If you have no love for self, how can you truly love anyone else? Everything starts with self. It is impossible to build anything outside of self if you have not yet built a solid foundation within yourself.

Before you can help in anyone else's healing process, you must first be healed. Forgiveness leads to Healing. Forgiveness is therapeutic. Therapeutic- adjective Relating to the healing of disease. - Oxford languages

As I've shown, unforgiveness acts as a disease. It acts as a disease because it affects us physically, mentally, and spiritually. Disease- noun A disorder of structure or function in a human especially one that has a known cause and a distinctive group of symptoms, signs, or anatomical changes. - Oxford languages

Once we identify the disease of unforgiveness in our lives, we must attack and address the root of the problem. We must align ourselves with a support group, life coach, church, Masjid, or whatever other resource or tool that will promote the process of healing. It may be a road of trial and error before we find out what actually works for us. Such goes life. There is no exact science because everyone and every case is unique. "And verily, whosoever shows patience and forgives that would truly be from the things recommended by Allah- The Noble Qur'an Surah 42:43

It is natural for us to want to be pleasing in God's sight. So, the Surah suggests that for us to be pleasing, we must therefore be patient and forgiving. We know that it is pleasing because the Surah states that it is recommended by God. So, if it is recommended, it, therefore, must be pleasing for patience and forgiveness to be recommended. If this is indeed the case, then God's recommendation ultimately would be for us to be patient with ourselves and others and forgiving to ourselves and others.

Why patience?
Because the process does not happen automatically. It is not a quick fix or instant transformation. It can be a long road, but the road leads to peace, love, and happiness. It is definitely a road worthy of travel. If patience is applied, the payoff would be tremendous. Practicing patience promotes a calming effect amongst its host.

Why patience?
Because it is possible that along the road to healing, a person may get frustrated. A person may get overwhelmed which causes them to revert to old habits. It is humanistic to have lapses, especially in the early part of the journey. A person may backslide, but that does not remand them to the obscurities of being a failure. This is why patience is necessary. As stated earlier it takes hard work, repetition, and continuity. It takes a true commitment. Time is crucial to change, and time is equivalent to patience.

So, as we see on the road to healing, we have to be patient, and with that patience, we must exercise forgiveness. Patience and forgiveness go hand-in-hand. One truly does not exist without the other.

Why forgiveness?
All human beings at one time or another have committed an offensive act towards another by way of either word, thought, or deed. Over time, or in some cases instantaneously, we feel a need to be forgiven for our offensive acts and transgressions. This sets the stage for atonement and reparation. It ideologically works as a bridge that is needed in order to get to the other side. Forgiveness allows us to cross over into the realm of atonement and reparation. We cannot be forgiven if we don't forgive, won't forgive, or can't forgive.

"One who does not know to forgive, should not expect to be forgiven".
 -Swahili proverb

14" For if you forgive men their trespasses, your heavenly Father will also forgive you. 15" But if you do not forgive men their trespasses, neither will your Father forgive your trespasses". Nkjv Matthew 6:14-15

It is likened to wanting something for nothing. You want the gift of forgiveness but don't want to give it in return. It doesn't work that way. Forgiveness is a two-way street. Bottom line it is reciprocal. The act of forgiveness to either someone else or to self serves as a liberator. This act frees us from the bondage of anger, disappointment, and all the negative energies associated with unforgiveness. This one act is so powerful that if used with good intentions, it covers a multitude of discord that can be generational, tribal, or deeply embedded within our most inner sanctuary of self.

The ultimate forgiveness of self is paramount to living at our highest level of existence. If you can forgive yourself for self-transgressions, then you will be able to forgive others for transgressions against you. It works inward out. You must give in order to receive. You must give in and surrender to the thought of forgiveness. Furthermore, if you can give forgiveness to self, then to others, the balance would be that you will be able to receive someone's forgiveness towards you. That's the equality of the whole thing in a nutshell.

Self-forgiveness tears down walls of complacency, shame, fear, and mediocrity. It crashes through glass ceilings of worthlessness, guilt, and blame. The power of self-forgiveness cuts the restraints that tend to hold us back because of it. It frees us and allows us to soar to great heights. It's similar to a bird finally being released after years of a menial existence in a cage. Simply put It's freedom!

So, on the road to healing, we must continually exercise patience and forgiveness. When we revert to old habits and backslide, not only must we be patient with self and others, but we must also be forgiving of self and others. If we aren't then the negative components will destroy us. All of the hard work that we put in would be for naught. We must have the memory of an elephant.

We must remember that we are kings. We must remember that we are Queens. We must remember that we are winners. We must remember that we are worthy, blessed, and driven. We must remember that most of all we are forgiven. This must become our new mantra. This will become the key to our success. The ultimate type of forgiveness is forgiveness of self. Self-forgiveness is the ultimate. It is the necessary component required in order to heal.

When I was a child, I talked like a child, I thought like a child, I reasoned like a child. When I became a man, I put the ways of childhood behind me.

1 CORINTHIANS 13:11

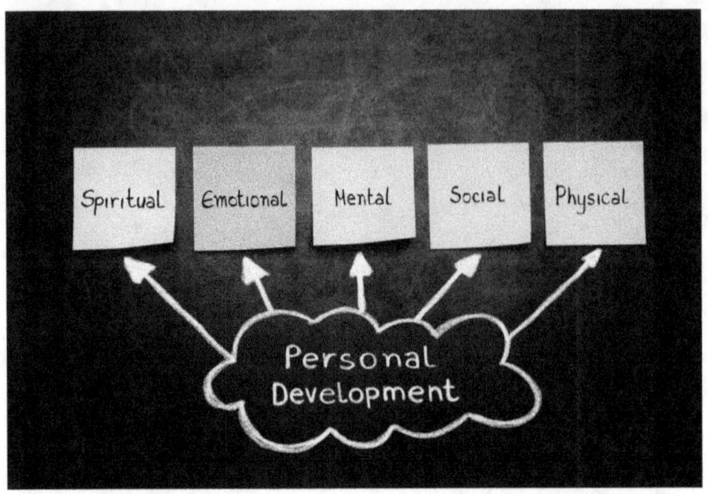

Forgiveness Comes With Maturity

During this talking point(Forgiveness comes with maturity), I'm going to pull from my own life experiences. I was born the only child to my mother and father. I have four other siblings from my mother. My father was 16, and my mother was 22 when I was conceived. She already had three other children at the time. Needless to say, she had her hands full. Four children, three different fathers, and several abusive relationships, and she suffered from depression and migraines. Toxicity was her norm.

At the age of around 6 months, my grandparents (from my father's side) took charge of me. They provided a stable and nurturing atmosphere. For that, I will forever be grateful. It was there that I grasped the concept of family, unity, love, and loyalty. Growing up in the early years I didn't see my father that much. When I did see him, it was mainly to discipline me for my behavior at school. Let's just say that I was a handful in school. My grandparents had grown weary of running back and forth up to P.S.45 for parent teachers' conferences. It was decided when I was twelve unbeknownst to me that I would go live with my father and stepmother.

Stubbornly I went because I didn't have a choice in the matter. I was told that I was going just for the summer. The summer was uneventful, and I missed home something awful. The school year fastly approached. I was looking forward to going to Junior High School with all of my childhood friends. Then the bomb was dropped on me. BOOM!!!! I wasn't going back to my grandparent's house. I was there to stay. This completely devastated me. My world was turned upside down. My new world now resided in Coney Island Brooklyn during the height of the crack epidemic.

No family was spared in C.I. during this epidemic. The fallout was catastrophic. It touched all of our households to some degree. My family was no exception, it hit us very hard too. My father had turned into a full-fledged "rockstar." He was totally consumed with crack cocaine. There were times when he didn't even go get his dialysis treatment. He was too busy beaming up to Scotty. I saw and felt the effects firsthand. Twelve years old, this was my introduction to the life.

It had gotten to the point where we eventually got evicted from housing. At this point, I was 14 years old mind you, and had become extremely embarrassed. I had become the butt of everyone's jokes. All of the taunting and teasing were directed toward me, The Crack Baby. I didn't want to show my face anywhere. Again I began to act out by disrupting school. It wasn't because I couldn't do the work, the work was easy. Unfortunately, that's how I chose to deal with my reality. My coping mechanism was to disturb the peace.

We eventually moved to Corona Queens. A new start with a clean slate. My father determinedly worked his way back to sobriety. In the last talking point, I discussed that you should align yourself with a support group, life coach, church, masjid, etc. Well, that's exactly what my father did.

He joined a church, gained a position, and developed the necessary faith needed to overcome. Looking back I wish to salute my father for achieving such an amazing feat. The odds were stacked against him. Unfortunately, most people don't outlive their addictions. Sadly most die enslaved in the state of addiction. He did not, when he died he was free and at peace. Salute.

So the combination of being tricked into living with my father, and the shame that his addiction cost me, caused me to develop a disdain for him. Even with him attaining sobriety, I could not jump over the hurdle of forgiveness. It always lurked in my heart, and it prevented me from having a closeness to him. Looking back it seems petty, but that's how I felt as a youth. I discussed this with someone before and was told at least I had a father. There's a thought. That I should be thankful regardless.

I carried a feeling that developed in my childhood well into adulthood. It was a feeling that was created in my immature mind. The feeling subconsciously lingered there. It created a wall between him and me. As I grew older I forgot all about why I felt the way I felt about him. I only knew that I felt a certain way. Disdain. Immaturely I had developed a feeling, held on to the feeling, and did not even remember why I felt that way. The reality changed, but the old immature feeling remained the same.

At home, I always felt uneasy. I vowed to leave as soon as I could. I graduated from Queens Vocational High School after getting expelled from August Martin. After graduation, I promptly joined the military. Still running, and searching for myself, I discovered that the military wasn't for me. I was honorably discharged, and I about-faced down another path. It was the same path that nearly destroyed my father. I immersed myself deeply in the street life. Before I knew it, I was totally addicted. Unbeknownst to me at the time, I carry the same addictive personality trait that my father carried.

My addiction however was the flip side of the coin from his addiction. He was addicted to using at one point, and I had become addicted to fast money and all that comes with that lifestyle. I thought that I was better, but I've since learned that addiction is addiction. One addiction is no worse or more prestigious than the other.

Needless to say with the fast life there are only two outcomes. The wise saying tells that you either end up dead, or you end up in prison. I was no exception to the rule. In life, you have choices, decisions, and consequences based on your actions. My decisions caused me the consequence of receiving 20 years in prison.

" Every man must decide whether he will walk in the light of creative altruism, or in the darkness of destructive selfishness".- Martin Luther King Jr

I operated out of selfishness, and greed. That greed drove me to my darkest point. It was during these times, my darkest days, that I had my brightest epiphany. During the whole process of my trial, my father was right by my side every step of the way. Day by day the veil was being removed from my eyes and my heart. I was starting to see through more mature eyes. I was beginning to see how life could shape some of the decisions and choices we make.
I was starting to develop an empathetic understanding of my father. My situation showed me that we were kindred, we were family, and we shared the same soul. Now, I could see a 16-year-old child with grown-man responsibilities existing in Bedford Stuyvesant (Old Brooklyn) in the '70s. I could see a 16-year-old child with no education, no skills, and looming health issues.

I can now see a 16-year-old child who wasn't capable of being a father figure because he didn't possess the wherewithal to do so. I was beginning to have an understanding, and having an understanding is a great part of life. Having an understanding brings clarity to a situation.

It was that clarity that helped me to see that having an addiction didn't make my father less of a man. That understanding helped to usher in the respect that I wasn't even aware didn't exist prior. I could now see that even in his turmoil, my father did what was best for me. He, along with my birth mother, allowed my grandparents to take charge of me. I could now see that this wasn't an act of abandonment. Just the opposite, it was an act of love. My eyes were wide open. I had gained an understanding, which brought about clarity, which created maturity.

I no longer thought of as a child. I no longer reasoned as a child. I no longer allowed the disdain that I developed in an immature mind to exist within me. I had put away childish thoughts. I had put away childish things. Maturity now dwelled in all the places where immaturity ruled. Growth and development were alive and well within me. This growth and development made way for a healthy relationship between my father and me. Before his transition, we had great dialogue and we were in a good place. I am so thankful for that opportunity.

Forgiveness can only come about with maturity. Maturity is the vessel that brings about forgiveness. The byproduct of maturity is developing an understanding. Once the understanding is understood, forgiveness can be made. There isn't an exact time frame for this to happen. You cannot base your time frame on someone else's time frame. You just have to put in the work. In due time maturity and forgiveness will develop. Forgiveness indeed comes with maturity.

"If a man who views the world the same at 50 as he did at 20 he has wasted 30 years of his life." -Muhammed Ali

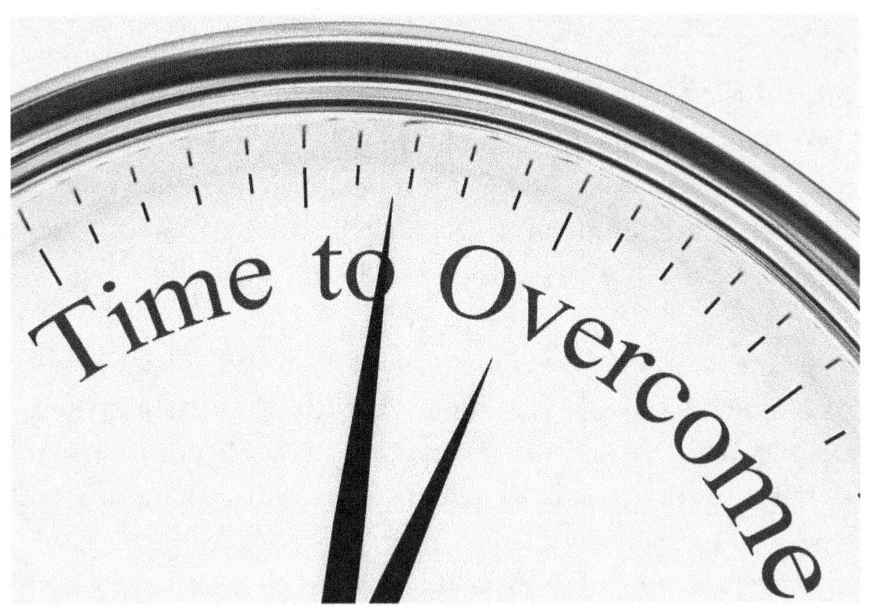

Overcoming

"Success is to be measured not so much by the position that one has reached in life as by the obstacles which he has overcome"
- Booker T Washington

People place value on a myriad of different things. How much money one may have, how popular one has become, how many likes they have received on the 'gram- some even place value on flashy jewelry or the name of their clothes. All of these things are vain and fleeting. They depreciate because these types of things change with the season. They are fickle, and they are not long-lasting.

Value should be placed on the things that serve to help shape our character. Things like life experiences that serve as obstacles, and the things that help us overcome them. We should value strength, perseverance, fortitude, patience, and of course forgiveness. These are the tools needed in order to assist us in overcoming said obstacles. These are the things that help shape and mold our character. The tools of strength, perseverance, fortitude, patience, and forgiveness are things that add value to our lives. It is a non-deprecatory type of value.

Without these tools, every time an obstacle arises in our lives, it will crush us. Without these tools we will feel defeated, worthless, dejected, and powerless. We will not be able to overcome anything in our lives. More importantly, we won't even be able to overcome ourselves. We will not be equipped to do so.

In order for us to become a person of substance, we must be able to overcome ourselves. Remember everything starts with self. We must start with overcoming negative self-reflection. We must overcome the fear that is attached to the quitter's mentality. We must overcome self-doubt. In order for us to be successful, we must overcome all of the excuses we tend to make as to why we are in the condition that we are in.

In order for us to overcome, we must gradually replace our mindsets from can't do, to can do. We must change our thoughts. If we are to truly overcome obstacles, then we have to change the view that we have of ourselves. The insecurity complex must be completely dismantled.

"Is it not written that ye are gods? I have said that ye are gods" - John 10:34. The vision of self must change indeed. "I said ye are gods. You are all sons of the Most High."- Psalms 82:6

If we view ourselves through this lens, then we will transition ourselves to greatness. It will assist us in seeing our worth.

The true test will be when the new storms arrive. When they do, we must be able to withstand them. Those are the times when we must batten down the hatches, and re-tap into the energy that helped to elevate us in the first place. We must remember continuity, repetition, and focus. After you have done all you can, just stand. This will be the start of you overcoming.

You can, you will, and you must. The healing process gives us the fortitude that we will rely on in our continued journey of life. Life's storms are the basic training that is needed in order to measure ourselves. It keeps us on point, and it restrains us so that we don't take on the air of arrogance. Storms also serve to strengthen our confidence. Embrace the storms of life, they should be viewed as a positive.

Once we see that overcoming is possible, we won't be so swift to revert back to our former selves. There will be no need to run and hide. There won't be any need to crumble, and there will be no need to panic. You can walk in the spirit of reassurance with confidence knowing that you will be able to withstand. This reassurance will bring about boldness in you. You will become unflappable, immovable, and empowered. The power to overcome is yours. It is within you. Believe it. Receive it. And live it!

-D.Shahid

.

"Forgiveness is a gift you
give yourself"

TONY ROBBINSON

Part 2
Trust The Process

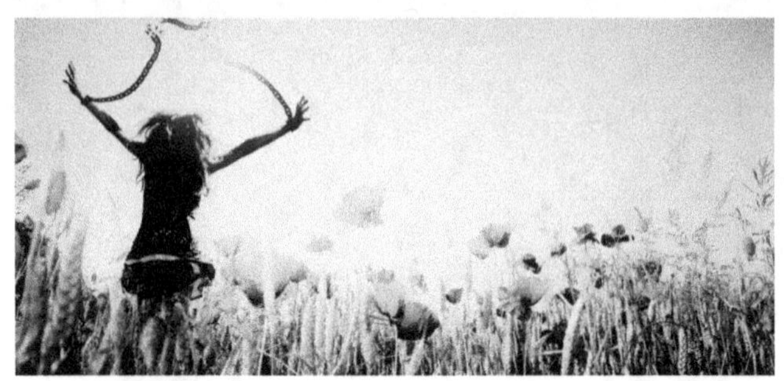

The Journey To Forgiveness

My journey to forgiveness was a long and daunting road. Bearing the burden of unforgiveness created resentment and anger that practically took over my body. When the anger finally became overwhelming, I began to reflect on my life, searching for an answer that could possibly give me some resolve. I needed clarity, any little thing that might give me a sense of peace. So many things happened in my life that contributed to the anger, I knew that for this healing process, it would be necessary for me to get to the root of the anger. So, I begin to ask myself a series of questions. Starting with, "Who am I most angry with?" The answer... My father. "Why am I so angry with him?" was my next thought. And for that question, I had to dig deep and allow myself to go into a very vulnerable space to find an honest answer.

The answer prompted some extremely deep self-talk, "When you were 8 yrs. old, he left our family for another woman; you were left alone to watch your mother unravel and become broken beyond repair." "You watched as he made that family priority, putting you second and not giving a damn how any of this would affect you." "You watched him only be concerned with what was going on in his household and have absolutely no concern for how his actions impacted the home he left, the home you lived in!" "And on top of that, he left his family for a woman that he knew would blatantly not accept you or your brother. As a matter of fact, you witnessed her attack him because she found out that he bought you something." "No one was there for you emotionally." "You felt like your mother didn't like you!" "You felt abandoned and unimportant to your parents."

"Of course you're angry. Who wouldn't be?!" OOOHHH! That was a lot to unpack!

I realized that as I lived life as an adult, I begin to manifest what I was feeling as a child. The resentment grew. The more it grew the more I manifested things into my life that made me feel abandoned and insignificant. Eventually, I turned into a very angry adult. After asking myself the hard questions and digging up all my childhood pain, the anger became even heavier and more draining. I eventually got tired of carrying it. I decided it was time to take the next step on my journey to forgiveness. I knew that this would require me to not only take a path of releasing resentment and anger but also forgiving more than just my parents. I would be required to forgive anyone that I ever felt wronged me. Initially, in my mind, I said, "That's never going to happen, I can't let anyone get away with doing me wrong". I later learned that these thoughts are a natural part of the process. And there are two reasons why. Number one, when you decide to make changes in your life you go through the 5 stages of the cycle of change: Stage 1 contemplation, stage 2 planning, stage 3 taking action, stage 4 maintenance, and stage 5 is relapse. When you have those "I want to let go, but I can't let them get away with that" thoughts you are entering the first stages of the cycle of change (contemplation). It's very easy to get stuck at this stage.

I battled with my thoughts for many years before I decided enough was enough. The reason why it's so easy to get stuck at this stage when you're attempting to start the forgiveness process leads me to the second reason why the "I want to let go but I can't let them get away with that" thoughts are a natural part of the process. And that is because, in the begging of the forgiveness phase, forgiveness could feel as if you're letting the person that wronged you off the hook. Forgiving someone who has hurt you doesn't mean you're letting that person off the hook. It doesn't mean you're completely healed from what they've done to you. It simply means you are letting go of the emotional baggage. Forgiveness isn't about letting the person off the hook, it's about letting yourself off the hook.

People also sometimes get the misconception that if you are forgiving you are also forgetting, or excusing the harm done to you. We've all been told at one point in life to "Forgive and forget." FYI that is horrible advice! Why? Well, in most cases forgetting is impossible, and even unhealthy. In order for someone to forget, it would usually involve suppressing emotions and thoughts caused by the harm/offense, and moving forward without processing what happened, or having the opportunity to express their feelings. It's much healthier to process stressful or harmful experiences. To do that you must lean into your emotions, thoughts, and conclusions that you've drawn about the experience and yourself, which is the total opposite of forcing yourself to "try" to forget the experience. Processing your emotions requires you to identify and label the feelings that are brewing. Give yourself the time and space to feel how you feel without judgment. With processing it's much easier to move into a space of healing.

So, it's time to break our generational cycles, change the unhealthy way of thinking and seek healthy and productive ways to heal. Let's face it, true personal healing and forgiveness can be a difficult thing to do and has no timeline. There are some things you can never forget, but you can forgive. We are now letting go of the expectations to "forgive and forget". Forgetting has nothing to do with real forgiveness. We are now moving to a place of healing by encouraging others to process their emotions and experiences, and then begin to forgive.

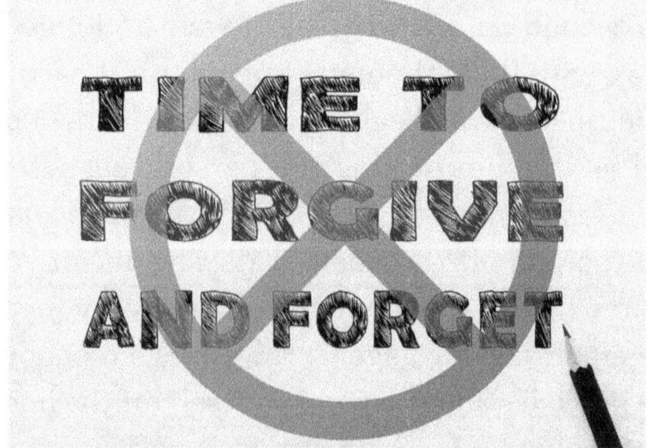

The most impactful lesson on my forgiveness journey was learning that I could get closure without involving the person that hurt me. Forgiveness is something you do without any response from the person who offended you. Your closure should not be dependent on the actions of the offender. This usually includes wanting, or expecting an admittance of wrongdoing or an apology. I can recall having a conversation with my mother about some of my experiences as a child that hurt me and affected my life. She was receptive and apologetic. I thought that an apology would have a big impact on my healing process, but the truth of the matter was that an apology was honorable, but it didn't take away the pain. My father was a different story, I knew that he would never take responsibility for his actions, nor would I ever get an apology. The conversation with my mother taught me that I didn't need an apology to heal. What I needed was to take responsibility for my healing journey by choosing to forgive, and making the decision to let go of the hurt.

"Your healing journey is yours, and yours alone. If you are waiting for someone to change, apologize, or take responsibility for their actions to start a healing journey, there's a good chance you'll never get started."
– Dr. Tandy

Choosing to forgive, and accept my parents for who they were, looking at my difficult and hurtful moments as lessons, and turning my life experiences into tools that I could use to be a better me as I move forward in life, have been the most empowering part of my forgiveness journey. Forgiveness bought me peace that allowed me to focus on myself and move on with my life.

There's nothing more effective for healing deep wounds than forgiveness. Throughout my forgiveness journey, I discovered 5 important components of forgiveness that I would like to share with you. Take time to reflect on how you can apply this to your journey.

Figure out what forgiveness looks likes to you.
Forgiveness can look different at each phase of the journey, and at different times of the journey, it is necessary for your overall mental wellness. If it is carrying baggage from your childhood like I did, or holding on to resentment, forgiveness is a process that takes time, and you get to decide what that process means to you. You are in charge of how to approach the process. Figure out what is most comfortable for you. It could be writing a letter, saying a prayer of forgiveness, or simply talking to the person about what hurt you and why it hurt you. Remember choosing forgiveness is choosing to heal.

Connect with your inner child.
To begin healing you must first acknowledge the presence of your inner child. This means recognizing and accepting the things that caused you pain as a child. Bringing this pain that we tuck away out of that dark space, will help you understand the impact that it has had on your life. Pay close attention to the feelings that come up and how you may be triggered by these emotions as an adult. Journal about your painful childhood experience from an adult perspective. Offer insight that you didn't understand as a child. In some situations, this could help you see the experience in a different light. It may even begin to make sense. Sharing these revelations with your inner child could make forgiveness an easier process.

Find purpose in your pain.
It is important to find meaning in your pain. Without meaning you lose your sense of purpose, which can lead to hopelessness and despair. Look at ways your suffering has changed you in a positive way.

As I stated earlier, I used my pain as a lesson and looked at the tools I developed to get through those difficult moments. I begin to think about how I could use those tools to empower my forgiveness journey. I became even more resilient. I even felt fearless. I also began to change my perspective on life. I could clearly see what was needed to accomplish my goals.

Don't be mistaken. I never minimized my pain. Again, the key is to address the wounds, care for the wounds, and acknowledge the experience. If not, forgiveness will be a journey that feels impossible to start.

How do you find meaning in pain you ask? Well... start by focusing on serving others. I realized that the pain and suffering that I endured, was so that I could show others how to grow from their pain. I also found meaning in speaking my truth, sharing my experiences in a space of healing, and empowering others. Founding Redesign Your Life, LLC was my purpose and direction in my forgiveness journey. "Within your pain lies your purpose." -Dr.Tandy

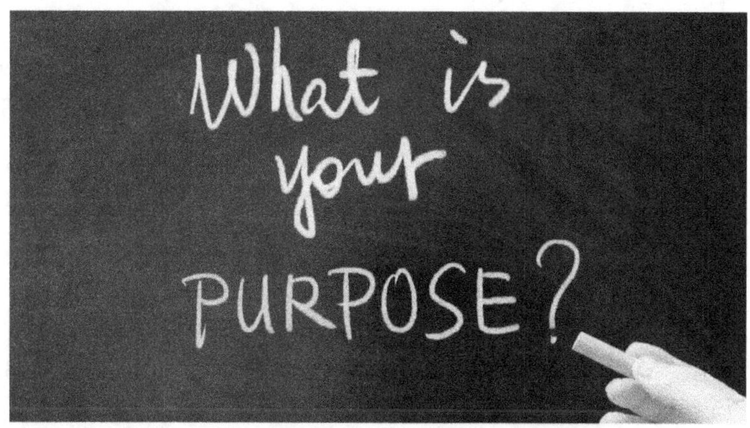

Practice, Practice, Practice.

Forgiveness is not an overnight process, it takes practice. Just like any other routine you have to build your forgiveness heart slowly. You have to implement your forgiveness tools into your everyday life on a regular basis. Make conscious decisions not to talk negatively about yourself, people that have hurt you, or your hurtful experiences. Refraining from negativity will nourish the forgiving side of your mind and heart. Practice showing love and compassion, recognize the uniqueness in everyone and be kind in your everyday encounters. Pouring love and light into every space you step in will help you to create a forgiving heart.

When forgiving is too hard, get help.

Forgiveness is always hard. Some people will never be able to let go of resentment and anger refusing to start a forgiveness journey. And that's ok! We are all on a personal timeline. However, if you want to forgive, but just can't figure out how to let go of the resentment and anger, or how to address the pain, surround yourself with wise people who support you, and get help. Consider talking to a therapist, hiring a coach, or think about using alternative methods. Energy healing is a powerful alternative method that has been responsible for taking my healing journey to another level. Emotion Code, Body Code (energy healing), and Hypnotherapy are the two methods that I found most effective for me (there are many different options to choose from). The results had such a powerful impact on my life that I was compelled to add these techniques to my practice. You can read my book "The Diva Code" if you're interested in learning about the energy healing techniques that I am certified in. You can also educate yourself on unprocessed emotions and negative energy that can block you from forgiveness, love, and happiness, and have an effect on your body.

Remember, if you are struggling that doesn't mean you are failing. Forgiveness is a process that takes time, practice, and determination.

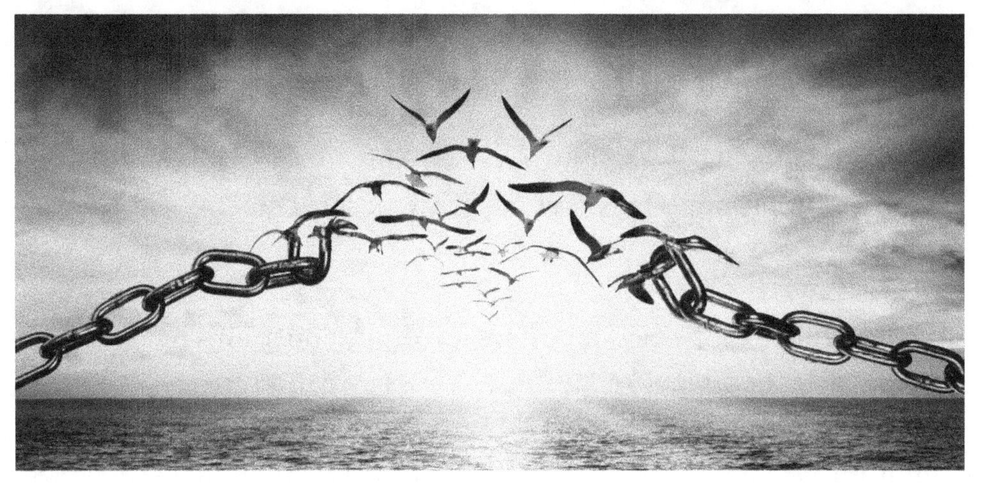

The Power Of Forgiveness

My clients often ask me "Why should I forgive?" My response is the same every single time: "If you want to heal, what are your other options?" As I've said many times, forgiveness is not to undo the damage, it gives you the opportunity to move forward in your life free from the negative effects of anger and resentment. To understand the power of forgiveness, you must first clearly understand what forgiveness is.

What is forgiveness?
Forgiveness means different things to different people. But in general, it involves an intentional decision to let go of resentment and anger.

The experiences that hurt you might always stay with you, but working towards forgiveness will lessen the grip that it has on you. It can help free you from the control that the emotions have over your life. Sometimes, forgiveness might even lead to feelings of understanding, empathy, and compassion for the person who hurt you. Healing could be a never-ending process. More often than not, it turns out to be an open-ended journey.

Forgiveness is a powerful force. It can transform, heal, deliver, repair, elevate, bless, and empower anyone. It's so powerful that it influences relationships, personal growth, self-esteem, and overall well-being.

Forgiveness transformed all of my anger and hurt into healing and peace. The bondage of unforgiveness was so heavy, that I developed anxiety, and was taking prescribed meds to control it. Thankfully, it was the power of forgiveness that helped me to overcome the anxiety. Turning my anger and hurt into healing and peace allowed me to let go of the hurt, disappointment, anger, and resentment that started from the feelings of abandonment by my father and two failed marriages.

No doubt, this healing process took a lot of work, a lot of contemplating, and a lot of reflecting. Reflecting was an essential part of this process. During my reflection time, I asked myself a series of questions. These questions prompted deep thought that led me to profound answers that provided so much clarity. I learned that the clarity was necessary, it allowed me to clearly see in which direction I needed to take this journey. Below are the reflection questions that were most helpful for me. Before asking yourself the questions, relax and take deep breaths. Take time to connect with your higher self, then dig deep for your answers.

First, ask yourself.
What hurtful experiences am I currently holding on to? Am I wanting the person to somehow pay for the pain they caused? How does this make my heart feel?

After you get the answers.
Dr. Tandy's coaching recommendation: Forgive; release the need to see the person experience pain or suffering; that job belongs to the universe.

Now ask yourself.
Why am I determined to not forgive this person? Am I carrying the weight of unforgiveness, and harboring bitterness towards this person?

After you get the answers.
Dr. Tandy's coaching recommendation: Let it all go and forgive them, it's not worth destroying your heart.

This might sound crazy, but forgiveness is not about how you feel. At the end of the day, you may never feel like starting the journey of forgiveness. But you know what? Forgiveness is a choice to stand in your power that you make from determination, not your emotions. Be ok with asking for forgiveness. Learn to forgive others, and choose to forgive yourself. Forgiveness is a choice and an act of empowerment.

Forgiveness is an important process. If not for others, for yourselves. The ability to accept and move on from bottled-up emotions of anger and resentment can be a healthy habit. While we all do it in our own time, finding and implementing the tools that work for you is important. Understanding the importance of self-forgiveness, and being able to routinely exercise forgiveness is essential to your well-being, mental wellness, and healing process. Staying in anger and resentment will only manifest additional emotional pain.

Lean In to Forgiveness

Write the name of the person you need to forgive:

What feels good about not forgiving this person?

What do you potentially lose in your life if you do not forgive this person?

Which of your important relationships will be in jeopardy if you choose to forgive this person? Which relationships will be in jeopardy if you don't?

What was your part in the situation that caused your pain? What is your part in the painful situation now?

Is this unforgiveness taking up space in your mind and distracting you from things that matter to you?

Does this unforgiveness make you feel in control of something or someone? What? Who?

What will relinquishing that control feel like for you?

Write three things you are grateful for that are not in jeopardy with the choice to forgive or not to forgive.
1.
2.
3.

I accept responsibility for my part in this. I am love. Forgiveness is love. Nothing and no one has the power to c[hange] my character.

I choose to forgive, not because ___________________ is not at fault, but because we are both flawed hum[an] beings, and I deserve to be free.

I forgive ___________________, and I choose to move on from the fear and resentment that have stuck aro[und] long enough.

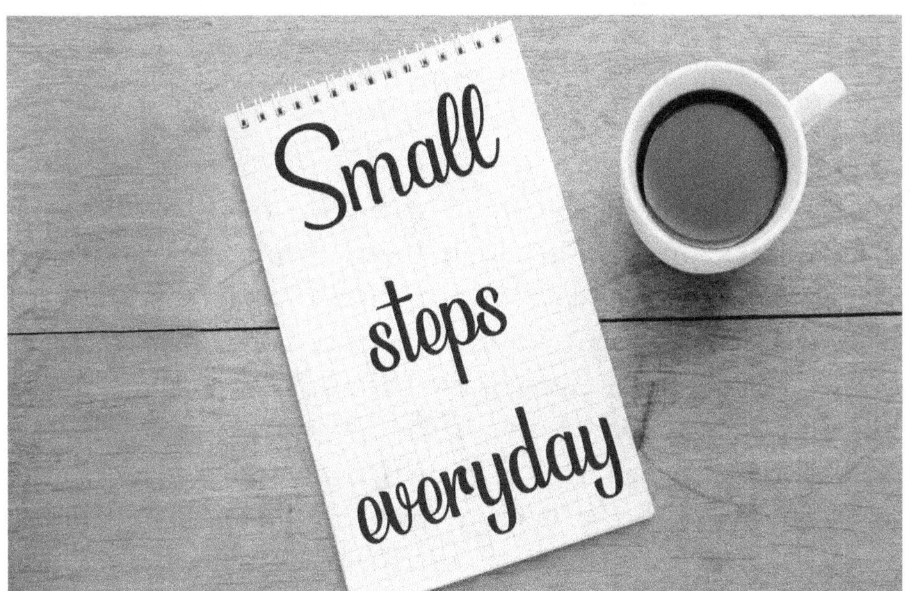

Taking The Steps To True Forgiveness

Forgiveness is a process of introspection and self-refinement. We forgive for the sake of our mental wellness. Holding on to the past is a heavy burden to carry. The longer we hold on to the past, the more power we give it. You owe it to yourself to move past hurtful experiences. These experiences do not determine who you are. Forgiveness is the process of change and is sometimes a difficult process.

This has been stated many times throughout the book only because we want to make it clear that the process will take putting in the hard work. Here is where I give you the tools to make the process a little smoother. Before I share my steps to forgiveness, did you know that it is 3 types of forgiveness and 4 phases of forgiveness? I wasn't aware of this until I began to study and research the complex concept of forgiveness.

So, first, let's talk about the 3 types of forgiveness.

Exoneration

We generally have this in mind when we think of the word forgiveness. Exoneration generally means wiping the slate clean and restoring the relationship to its previous state. It's the old saying we talked about earlier "Forgive and forget." When someone is exonerated, it's as if the harmful act never took place. As discussed earlier, part of the reason why it can be so difficult to forgive is that we believe forgiveness always means wiping the slate clean. Remember it doesn't always mean that, and the old saying is bad advice. However, there are 3 situations in which exoneration could be acceptable.

1.   **The hurtful act was an accident**. No fault or blame is applied to any party involved. We all make mistakes and sometimes the appropriate response is to forgive completely.

2.   **The person committing the wrongdoing is a child or someone who couldn't understand the implications of their actions.** In these situations, the person wronged has positive or loving feelings toward the person committing the wrongdoing.

3.   **The person who hurt you has true remorse and takes full responsibility for their actions.** No excuses, they ask for forgiveness, and after you feel confident that the hurtful action will not happen again you by choice wipe the slate clean.

Forbearance

This level of forgiveness applies when the wrongdoer makes a partial apology or lessens their apology because they feel that you are also partially to blame for their wrongdoing. They may even imply that you caused their actions. The apology usually doesn't feel authentic. It often sounds like "I'm sorry you feel that way" or "If I did anything that made you feel... I'm sorry."

Forbearance is usually the forgiveness usually applied when the relationship at hand is one that you are willing to work at. In this case, you should stop dwelling on the wrongdoing, let go of any grudges you hold, and all thoughts of revenge. Unlike exoneration, the slate is not wiped completely clean. Instead, with forbearance it's best to maintain a watchful eye over the wrongdoer. It's the old saying "Forgive but don't forget" or "Trust but verify." Forbearance is continuing the relationship but not fully trusting at the current time.

Most of the time forbearance is temporary. If the wrongdoer maintains good behavior for a desired time frame, they may earn back your trust. If so, forbearance could switch to exoneration. Of course, the time required for this to happen would totally be determined by you.

Release
This level of forgiveness applies to situations in which the wrongdoer has never acknowledged any wrongdoing. You receive no apology, or they offered an insincere apology. Even though it is hard to offer this type of forgiveness, you should in fact do so. This form of forgiveness is not continuing the relationship, but you let go of your negative feelings and any fixations on what happened to you. Release requires you to stop defining your life by the hurt done to you, and it allows you to let go of the burden. This burden erodes your ability to be happy and enjoy peace of mind.

Before moving on to the phases of forgiveness I want to reiterate, to fully forgive sounds nice but exoneration isn't always possible. And forbearance, "Forgive but don't forget" isn't always the right option depending on the circumstances and the relationship. But choosing not to let go of the past hurts you more than it will ever hurt the person who has wronged you.

Dr. Robert Enright was one of the pioneering researchers on forgiveness, and also the first to develop a comprehensive model of forgiveness. He began incorporating his ideas of forgiveness into his therapy sessions. Those who underwent therapy that had a focus on forgiveness saw greater improvements than those who didn't. Dr. Enright eventually came up with his model of forgiveness. The model is made up of four key phases.

Phase 1. The Uncovering Phase

Thinking about forgiveness first involves thinking about how exactly you were wronged and how has it affected your life. The Uncovering Phase means embracing, rather than avoiding, what has happened and what you are feeling. The goal is to be as objective as possible; you cannot begin to forgive unless you truly understand the events that triggered your hurt.

Phase 2. The Decision Phase

In this phase, you actively decide to start the process of forgiveness. Forgiveness must be a choice you make on your own. Sometimes, you choose to forgive because you realize that being angry and resentful doesn't serve you. Forgiveness becomes a real possibility with a positive outcome.

Phase 3. The Work Phase

In the work phase, you are actually putting in the work of forgiveness. This does not mean excusing an offense or necessarily reconciling with the offender. Instead, it means trying to better understand the wrongdoing from an objective side, to understand the motive or reasoning behind the wrongdoing. When you do this, you are more likely to see the wrongdoer as human rather than just a malicious force. It helps to recognize the wrongdoer as human this makes it easier to have compassion and empathy. In this phase, you not only accept the pain of what has happened but begin to let go of resentment and you may begin to have mercy.

Phase 4. The Deepening Phase

In this, the hard work is done. And you will start to see the effects of releasing negative emotions. You begin to clearly see the purpose of your pain and feel the burden of forgiveness become much lighter. In turn, you may also start realizing how you too may need forgiveness from others.

These four phases are only an overview of Dr. Enright's concept, they are designed to show you what forgiveness could look like in practice. Seeing forgiveness broken down as a process can offer you a clearer vision of what your healing can look like. We see that out of hurt comes hope. At the end of this section, there are four worksheets that will help you in your journey of each phase.

Before I move on to the steps of forgiveness, I want to briefly discuss mindset and forgiveness. One of the very first things I tell my clients in consultations is "Your brain will always take you back to what is comfortable and familiar". Why is this? Well, your subconscious mind has a great amount of control over your positive and negative thoughts, the key is to train your brain to produce more positive thoughts. This is where your conscious mind comes in. You can use your consciousness to reprogram or retrain your subconscious mind to do things that are more beneficial for your current and future life.

One method I show my clients to use that will help retrain the brain is affirmations. Affirmations have also helped me to reprogram my negative thoughts and beliefs.

I used what I call forgiveness affirmation to reprogram my beliefs on forgiveness and it made the process of letting go a little easier. So, on the following page, I have a list of affirmations that have helped me along the way.

Read these affirmations out loud and let the sound of your voice resonate in your heart and mind. As you say your positive affirmations, also spend time to visualize yourself releasing any negative thoughts, beliefs, and energy out and into the sky for the universe to dissolve. Repeat one or more of these affirmations every day. You can also say them while doing chores, driving, when you feel angry towards a person or situation, frustrated or sad. As you start to believe in these forgiveness affirmations, it becomes easier to forgive yourself and others.

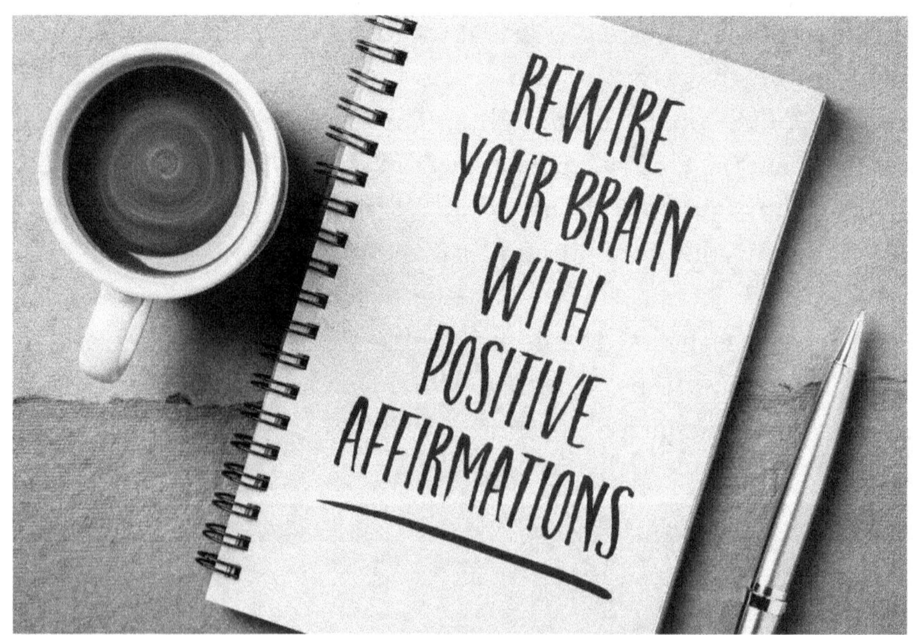

Daily Forgiveness Affirmations

I release my anger.

Negative energy is not welcome here.

I forgive people who hurt me although it is not an easy process when I feel hurt.

Forgiveness enables me to move forward to higher vibration.

I live joyfully in the now and design my future.

The past has no effect on my present.

I am anchored in my body and present in the moment.

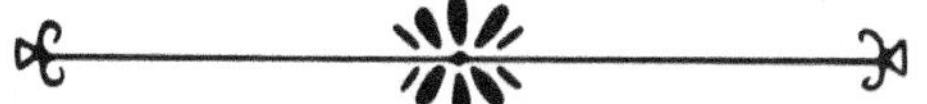

So, I have talked about the 3 types and the 4 stages of forgiveness, I gave you some positive affirmations, and I now want to help you start the journey by giving you my 6 steps to true forgiveness.

Step 1. Embrace your feelings.

Have you ever tried to convince yourself "That didn't bother me" or "I don't care" in response to a hurtful situation? And how did that work out for you? Resisting painful emotions is rarely ever effective. When you are hurt by someone's words or actions, it's important to acknowledge the pain and allow yourself to feel it. Don't beat yourself up for whatever emotions the experience caused. In time you will you'll be ready to put the situation into proper perspective. But while the feelings are there, embrace them.

At the same time, don't direct your energy to unnecessary negativity by reminding yourself of all the past wrongs this person has committed, or how this person "always" or "never" does something. Remember to stay in the moment.

Step 2. Analyze your emotions.

Analyze your emotions and how the hurt and pain have affected you. The word "analyze" is key here because it involves thinking before making a decision. Before you decide on whether or not you will forgive this person, consider the negative feelings you've experienced since the incident.

How has the pain changed you? How detrimental was the person's mistake to your life or someone else?

Step 3. Accept the situation.

Accept that you cannot change what has happened. No matter how hard you wish the situation and pain away, it's time to admit to yourself that the anger and resentment you are harboring punishes no one but yourself.

Step 4. Determine.
This is when the forgiveness process will either begin or end. It is during this step that you must think long and hard about what exactly you are considering forgiving and whether or not you want to forgive. Make it more about you than the other person so that you can take the last step and forgive!

Continuously ask yourself "How do I you feel"? Check-in with yourself and remember that life is short, and you are worth it to do the work.

Step 5. Find Ways to Let Go.
It is important to focus on the act of forgiving instead of allowing your feelings to get in the way. Focus on giving that person your forgiveness, even if your emotions make you feel like doing otherwise. I always suggest to clients, writing out the hurtful experiences to help release the poison of old pain. Writing out the pain helps increase emotional release. Also, sharing the hurtful experience with a trusted confidante, therapist, or coach provides significant relief.

Step 6. Forgive.
The act of forgiveness happens in your mind, it has nothing to do with the other person. This is where the past is left behind, pain is explored, and resolved so you can move on in life with peace and joy. You become more positive your mood is brighter and more hopeful. You are turning memories of painful past events into positive memories of healing and letting them go.

And now your children are raised in health and happiness, without destructive cycles from the past being replayed and passed on to future generations.

Forgiveness
Uncovering Phase

During the **uncovering phase** of forgiveness, you will improve your understanding of the injustice, and how it has impacted your life. Use the journal prompts below to begin exploring.

Describe the injustices you have endured. What happened? Why was this treatment unfair?

How have the injustices affected you? Circle any of the examples that apply, and describe them in the box below. Feel free to add something else that isn't listed.

painful emotions
(e.g. anger or shame)

changed behavior
(e.g. avoiding new relationships)

practical costs
(e.g. time or money)

changed worldview
(e.g. "people are evil")

cognitive rehearsal
(recurring thoughts about injustice)

physical harm
(e.g. injuries from abuse)

Forgiveness
Decision Phase

During the **decision phase** of forgiveness, you will gain a deeper understanding of what forgiveness is, and make the decision to choose or reject forgiveness as an option.

Without looking at a definition, how would you describe forgiveness?

Many people struggle with the decision to forgive because they know that they have the right to be angry, while the offender does not have the right to kindness. Making the decision to forgive means letting go of these resentments—which you have every right to hold—so you can heal.

What are the pros and cons of deciding to forgive the person who wronged you?

Pros	Cons

Whether or not you've made the decision to forgive, describe how things might be different if you decide to do so. Be as specific as possible.

Forgiveness
Work Phase

During the **work phase** of forgiveness, you will start to understand the offender in a new way, which will allow positive feelings toward the offender and yourself.

Learning to understand the offender, and to see them as more than their wrongdoing, is an important part of forgiveness. However, it must be stressed that understanding does not mean condoning. One can understand another person without believing their actions are acceptable.

Respond to one of the following prompts:
- **What was life like for the offender as they grew up? May this have impacted their behavior?**
- **What was life like for the offender at the time of the offense?**

List the feelings you currently have toward the offender.

Did you list any positive feelings toward the offender? If so, describe them. If not, describe how your negative feelings have changed over time. Have they lessened?

Forgiveness
Deepening Phase

During the **deepening phase** of forgiveness, you will further decrease the negative emotions associated with the injustice. You may find meaning in the experiences, and recognize ways in which you have grown as a result.

How have you benefitted by forgiving the offender? Consider how forgiveness has affected your emotional health, behavioral changes that resulted from the injustice, and time/energy spent thinking about the offender.

Describe how you have grown because of injustice you endured and your efforts to forgive. How has your worldview changed? Are you stronger than you were before deciding to forgive?

"The more you know yourself, the more you forgive yourself."

- CONFUCIUS

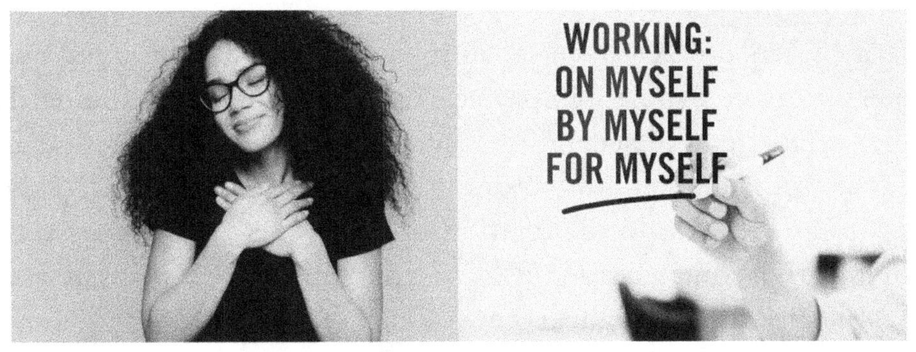

Self Forgiveness

The ability to forgive begins with the ability to forgive yourselves. Have you heard the saying "hurt people, hurt people"? We've all hurt someone at some point in life including ourselves. None of us are perfect. I don't know anyone that has led a perfect life or never needed to be forgiven for something they've said or done. We all make mistakes. But we tend to be harder on ourselves than we are on others. And the truth is, we need to offer to ourselves what we offer to loved ones who have hurt us, which is compassion and forgiveness.

There was a time that I needed a sense of inherent worth, despite my actions. For many years I was disgusted with myself for choosing my second husband. That choice came with so much trauma, misery, and pain and eventually brought a lot of pain and trauma to my son that affects him to this day. My son holds on to the anger refusing to let go or forgive. For me, it was easy to forgive my second husband. So easy that some years later my son asked me "How could you just move on like it never happened?" I had to! There was no way I was going to live 7 years of pure misery with someone, finally freeing myself from a dreadful situation, but still live in misery by holding on to my anger and resentment. I was glad to forgive him and move on. For me that was the easiest way not to ever have to look back. But what he didn't know was that I had the hardest time forgiving myself for allowing this pain and misery into our home.

What I learned was that in self-forgiveness, you honor yourself as a person, even if you are imperfect. I seriously broke my standards when I married my second husband. And I beat myself up for it. The self-punishment was draining, and I started to take a good look at how I got into the relationship, coming to some deep self-empowering conclusions that moved me towards self-compassion. It actually softened my heart toward me.

But you can easily get stuck in the story of what happened, and it could feel impossible to move past it. It damages your self-esteem and your willingness to take risks. The way you view yourself becomes slighted, filtered through the lens of "what you did wrong." Learning to forgive is about letting go of the guilt and shame. and that could be very difficult when you feel that you've hurt someone you love. I was carrying so much guilt and shame I felt as if I could not or should not forgive myself while my son was still hurting.

Shame will make you feel as if the experience of forgiveness, is like losing a part of yourself that deserves to suffer for what you have done. And self-punishment can become a way of life making it incredibly difficult to be able to see yourself as worthy of change.

Guilt breaks your spirits. For a moment, it may help to feel guilt after some self-reflection, but ultimately, you are human and in need of compassion. Guilt may make you feel like you are not enough, or worthy of forgiveness or love. And it prevents you from moving on with your life and becoming the best person you can be.

Starting today you are choosing to love yourself and consider yourself worthy even when you feel broken, especially when you feel broken. Everyone is worthy of love, and you are too.

Self-forgiveness Affirmations

I, (name), forgive myself completely.

I give up all shame now.

I release all guilt about past behavior.

I love myself enough to have compassion for my previous actions.

I did the best I could at that moment.

I am capable of moving beyond my mistakes.

I let go of all self-judgement and self-Sabotage.

I accept all of who I am.

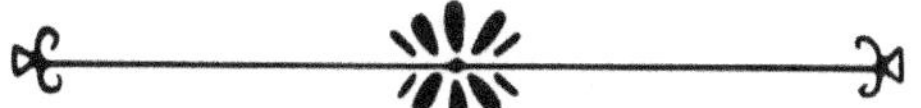

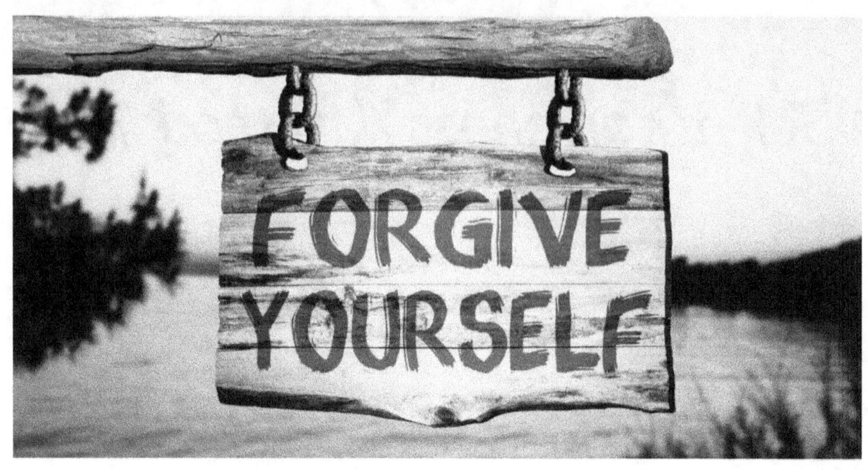

How To Start A Self Forgiveness Journey

We all make mistakes. But the key is to find out your why. The why will unlock your truth. You will know how you got to this point and make the important decision not to go down that path again.

Mistakes don't determine who you are or who you can become. It is not a reflection of your self-worth. So, how did I achieve self-forgiveness?

I unlocked the truth through the 4 R's of self-forgiveness. Responsibility, Remorse, Restoration, and Renewal.

Responsibility

Accept what happened while showing yourself compassion. This will help you avoid the self-destructive cycle of negative emotions.

Usually, this is done through self-talk or mentally and emotionally accepting what happened. Depending on the situation, this can be an acknowledgment that something was your fault or that it was not your fault.

Remorse

Second, embrace the negative feelings associated with responsibility. Whether it's letting go of guilt (the insidious sense that implies you're a good person who did something bad) or shame (the poisonous feeling that you are socially irredeemable), both need to be channeled into remorse.

Feelings of worthlessness, low self-esteem, depression, aggression, and, at worst, despair, can be lightened by allowing remorse to the surface. Feel the responsibility and you're halfway to self-forgiveness.

Restoration

This is the path you take to repair the damage that was caused. Start a healing journey. Seek support from friends, loved ones, or even a support group. We function best in groups where we feel accepted and supported by the people around us.

Renewal

Think of this step as your time to self-reflect. Taking a good look at what you did to understand why, and how you can avoid making the same mistake in the future. It is learning and growing to be better in the future. Renewal is the way to avoid self-hatred and prevent self-pity. It helps you continue the journey to self-healing and self-love.

If you continue to struggle with forgiving yourself and notice that your mental well-being is on a decline, seek help! There's no shame in needing professional help, and a therapist or coach will be able to guide you through the process of self-forgiveness.

SELF-FORGIVENESS

What was your mistake?

What emotions does this mistake make you feel?

What needs to be done for you to forgive yourself?

What have your learned?

What can you do differently next time if this
situation happens again?

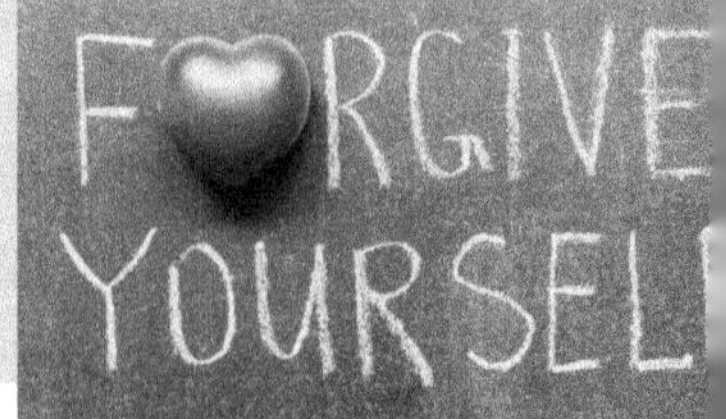

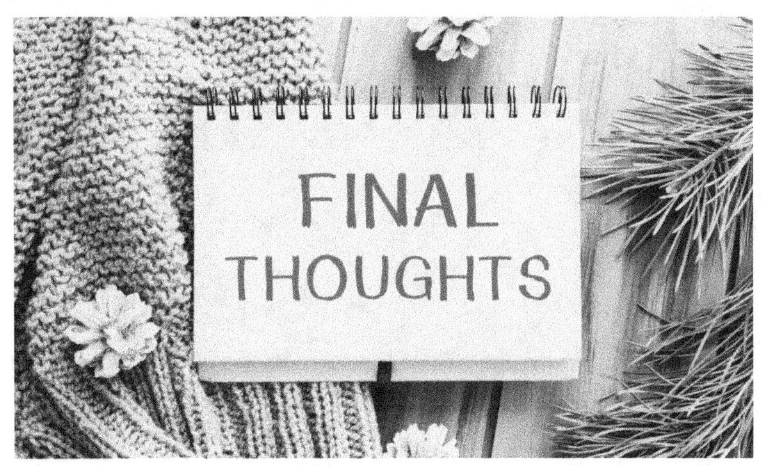

Forgiveness is about finding peace and joy in your life. Once you let go, you learn to live. It takes time, compassion for yourself, and the support of others to work through the pain. The resentment you hold on to when you fail to forgive others consumes your heart and damages your connection with the universe. When you withhold forgiveness, you are effectively putting a barrier up that keeps you from experiencing the power of connecting with your highest self.

Unforgiveness is like a cancer that eats away at the fibers of happiness, productivity, and a fruitful existence. Everything starts with self. Once we forgive ourselves, and others, the doors will open up and produce new thoughts. Those new thoughts are magnetic and are necessary for our elevation process. Without forgiveness and new thought, there will be no leveling up. One cannot exist without the other. They are dependent on each other.

 Repetitive thoughts have the power to manifest. The type of existence we have rests and lives in the thoughts we have. Mental maturity can and will produce the results that we visualize for ourselves. Once we develop in our level of maturity, we will be able to overcome our realities. It all begins with forgiveness. Forgiveness is emphatically therapeutic. -D. Shahid

21 Day Forgiveness Journal

"When you forgive you heal. When you let go you grow."

You've decided you're ready to forgive. Congratulations!

Forgiveness includes acknowledging that you are hurt, accepting the pain as your own, and being honest with yourself about the affect it's had on you. Forgiveness happens by being honest about what it was like for you to be betrayed, lied to, offended, mistreated, or abused.

Journaling is one of my favorite self-care activities and I encourage my clients to use it as a tool to learn to express themselves. Getting your thoughts from your head to paper is a great way to begin releasing feelings of unforgiveness. The negative thoughts connected to your pain/resentment can create a foggy mind and block you from living a peaceful life.

Change doesn't happen overnight, but a lot can happen in 21 days. Use this prompted journal every day for 21 days. Take time to reflect, put some real thought into journaling the answers to the questions. Answering the questions honestly and with deep thought will help you get a better understanding of what you're feeling and what steps you can take to overcome your hurt and move towards forgiveness.

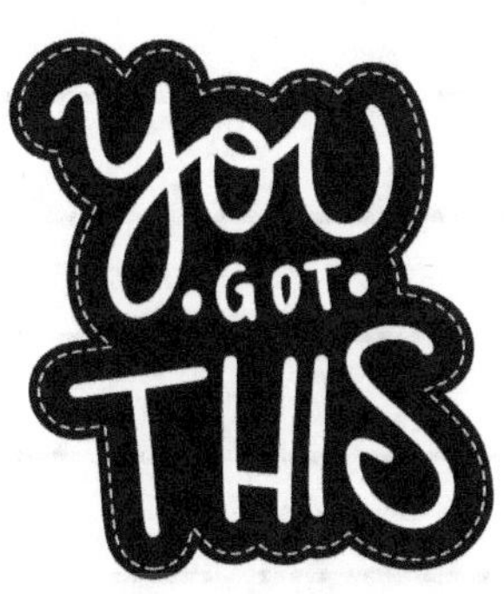

DAY

1

What experiences have you had with others that you believe you're still hurting from?

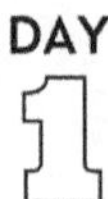

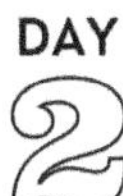

What does forgiveness mean to you?

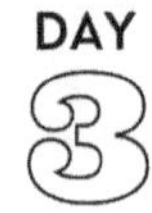

What are the benefits of forgiveness?

Do you need someone to say sorry to be able to forgive them?
Why?

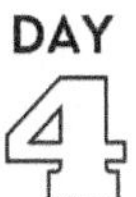

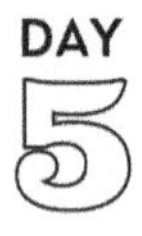

Who do you need to forgive and why?

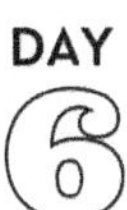

6

Do you find it easy to ask for forgiveness? Why? Why not?

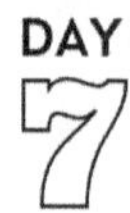

What do you need the most so you can forgive and let go?

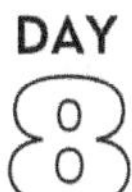

Name 4 things you can do today to help yourself feel good. Then write down a daily self-care routine to follow.

Are there any negative thoughts holding you back from forgiving?
What thoughts would you like to have instead?

10

What do you need to let go of that you have no control over?

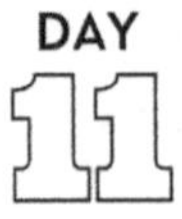

Do you think you've failed yourself in one way or another?

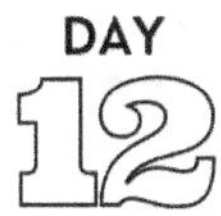

Do you have any regrets? What could you have done differently?

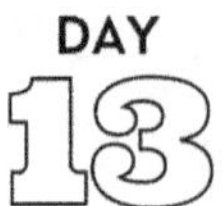

13

Do you examine your mistakes from a place of compassion or judgment?

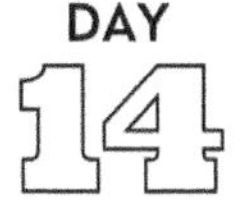

What do you need to forgive your younger self for not knowing?

How can your spirituality help you forgive?

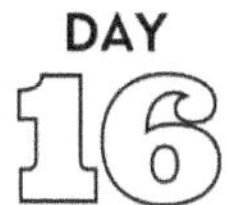

How can other people help you forgive and who can help?

Write down at least 8 affirmations for yourself related to forgiving yourself and others.

Example: Forgiveness is a gitf to myself
I accept my past and learn from it.

Speak These Affirmations Every Day For The Next 21 Days

How can your past empower you in the future?

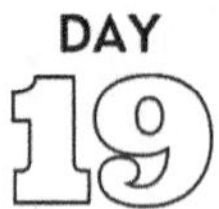

19

Write down some ways you can care for yourself physically, mentally, emotionally, and spiritually.

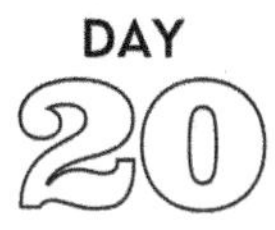

20

What are some new things you've learned about yourself from practicing forgiveness so far?

What do you still need to understand, or lack clarity about?

Notes

Notes

Notes